T0009822

# ALL
# YOU
# NEED
## IS REST

MITA MISTRY

ALL YOU NEED IS REST

An Hachette UK Company
www.hachette.co.uk

Vie Books, an imprint of Summersdale Publishers Ltd
Part of Octopus Publishing Group Limited
Carmelite House
50 Victoria Embankment
LONDON
EC4Y 0DZ
UK

www.summersdale.com

Printed and bound in China

ISBN: 978-1-80007-706-5

Substantial discounts on bulk quantities of Summersdale books are available to corporations, professional associations and other organizations. For details contact general enquiries: telephone: +44 (0) 1243 771107 or email: enquiries@summersdale.com.

# Contents

4 The Power of Rest

6 Welcome to Rest

31 Rest Your Mind

56 Rest Your Body

81 Welcome to Sleep

106 Sleep Self-Care

131 Good Nights

154 Conclusion

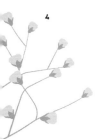

# THE POWER OF REST

In today's busy world there is an unspoken expectation to be on the go all the time, leaving many of us feeling like we can never truly unwind. Often, rest is considered to be indulgent and we can feel guilty taking a little time for ourselves. But rest is essential: how we relax, calm our minds and recharge our bodies directly impacts our well-being.

Most of us yearn to unplug from the world and let every cell in our body breathe a sigh of relief at the respite this offers. Thankfully, there are effective ways to bring those moments into even the busiest of days – and it's easy to do, once you know how.

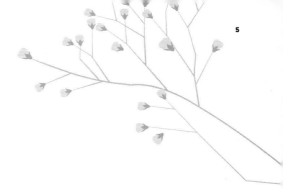

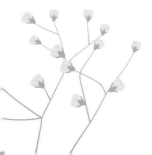

By learning about the different types of rest and following practical tips to help your mind and body, you will start to feel energized, happier and more relaxed across all areas of your life.

Rest has the power to recharge your ability to deal with the niggles of life, including in areas such as study, work or relationships, as well as to enhance your overall health. This book shows you how to do just that, so read on and tune in to the power of rest.

# Welcome to Rest

Rest is not the same as sleep. We might think getting enough sleep should meet all our restorative needs, but we require different types of rest in order to flourish. That's why some people still feel exhausted after a good night's slumber. Not getting enough rest can leave us feeling tired, stressed, overwhelmed or even burned out. But by understanding our needs, we can easily bring restorative moments into our day to give us that much-needed refresh. Read on to learn how.

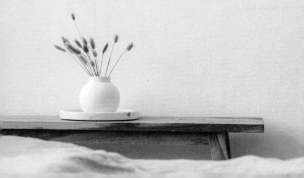

# GET ENOUGH REST

Science tells us that resting for 42 per cent of the day (10 hours of rest in various forms) is what our bodies require to function optimally. So if you struggle to get up at the weekend, it could be because your busy week is catching up with you.

If we don't rest enough, built-up stress can affect every function in our body, including our immune system, cardiovascular system, digestive functioning and hormones. Resting is essential to keep these processes healthy.

It might sound impossible, but fear not, you don't have to spend 10 hours with your feet up every day. Rest can be balanced over a week or even a month.

*If you get tired,*
*learn to rest,*
*not to quit.*

BANKSY

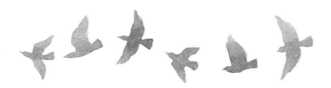

# REST MATTERS, YOU MATTER

Rest can look different for everyone – it's any behaviour which boosts physical or mental well-being, such as going for a walk or simply taking deep breaths. These daily actions improve mental health, lower stress and anxiety, reduce blood pressure, increase concentration and memory, strengthen the immune system, uplift moods and even enhance metabolism.

Rest matters, not just so that you're more efficient or able to juggle more, but because you deserve to be healthy, happy and to thrive. Plus, the people in your life deserve you at your best. The following pages tell you what different types of rest you might need.

# TUNE IN TO YOUR BODY

Niggling aches or pains could be a sign that your muscles are being overused – perhaps from standing or sitting for long periods – and you need some physical rest to recharge. Most people experience bothersome aches that are caused by daily life, especially if they sit at a desk, stand, walk or exercise for long durations. Perhaps you've noticed some discomfort in your shoulders from sleeping awkwardly. Physical relaxation can be passive, such as having naps, while active relaxation includes gentle stretches to improve your flexibility and circulation.

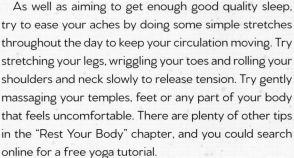

As well as aiming to get enough good quality sleep, try to ease your aches by doing some simple stretches throughout the day to keep your circulation moving. Try stretching your legs, wriggling your toes and rolling your shoulders and neck slowly to release tension. Try gently massaging your temples, feet or any part of your body that feels uncomfortable. There are plenty of other tips in the "Rest Your Body" chapter, and you could search online for a free yoga tutorial.

But if your aches last a long time, please see your doctor for more help.

# CREATE MENTAL BREATHING SPACES

Do you ever get brain fog or forget things because you're thinking about too much at once? If your mind races over thoughts of work or family when you're trying to sleep, or you feel your brain never switches off, you might need some mental breathing space.

Anything that gives your brain a break from intense thinking or focusing too much is helpful. Set reminders on your phone to stop, slow down and breathe for 3 minutes every 2 hours. Go for a walk or do something that requires little mental energy, like washing the dishes.

# Let your senses unwind

Life is noisy. From the moment we wake, most of us spend entire days engulfed in noise: the pinging notifications on our phones, the TV, people chattering and the traffic. It's not just our ears that are bombarded with input: we experience constant visual and olfactory stimulation too. Our senses are overwhelmed with everything from bright lights and glaring screens to the smells around us, so it's not surprising we often feel irritated or angered by this sensory overload.

Try unplugging from the world around you for a day so you can let your senses unwind. Use noise-cancelling headphones, turn off notifications, briefly close your eyes or avoid loud environments.

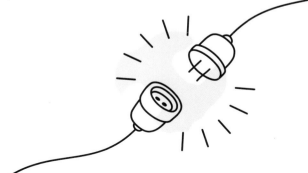

# REBOOT YOUR CREATIVITY

We face hundreds of choices every day – from what to wear or cook to more complex decisions about our work, family or study. Time spent problem-solving, thinking up new ideas and making daily decisions uses up our creative energy. It's hardly surprising that decision fatigue is real. Research shows we make our best decisions when we are rested.

Refill your creative reservoir by spending time exploring nature, appreciating the sunset and trees and absorbing art or beauty in any form. You might not see yourself as creative, but everyone is in some way and your creativity needs nourishing.

*Each person deserves a day in which no problems are confronted, no solutions searched for.*

MAYA ANGELOU

# TAKE A RESPONSIBILITY BREAK

Being responsible for our lives and those who depend on us is so important. But when the weight of our responsibilities starts to break us, we must recognize the signs and realize that it's okay to have time out before we completely crumble.

Most of the time, not everything needs to be completed or even decided the same day. Take time out from your responsibilities and when you return you will feel recharged and more able to tackle any problems.

What responsibilities can you put down for a little while so that you can relax and restore your strength?

# RESTORE MEANING

Sometimes we might feel like our work or life makes little difference, which can leave us feeling unfulfilled, exhausted and eventually burned out. We may not realize it, but deep down we all need to feel like we belong – it's a human instinct to feel that our efforts are somehow contributing to the greater good.

One way to connect to this desire is by engaging in activities that fill you with a sense of purpose, such as getting involved with a charity, community project or helping someone. Even small acts of kindness can leave you feeling more fulfilled.

# Have a social sanctuary

Most of us spend time with people who deplete our energy – friends, co-workers or family members who constantly need something from us. It's not that they're terrible human beings or that we don't care, it's just that sometimes we need a break from people who are always asking us for something.

A good social network is the number-one predictor of happiness, and this is where social sanctuary comes in. It means spending time with people who support you and bring out the best in you, leaving you feeling more energized than before.

A social sanctuary offers meaningful interaction and the freedom to be your utterly wonderful self without the fear of disapproval.

One way to figure out if you need a social sanctuary is to ask yourself when you last spent time with people who didn't need anything from you.

Seek out social sanctuary: have a meaningful chat with your partner (set a 30-minute timer to discuss your days), go on a walk with a friend or have a coffee with someone who makes you feel positive and fulfilled.

# LET YOUR EMOTIONS REST

Most of us hold on to our emotions, either to please people or simply because we feel unable to express them, but this uses up a lot of energy and is exhausting. When you don't have the freedom to be truly authentic about your feelings, it can leave you numb, angry, lashing out at people or full of self-doubt.

In contrast, when you're in a safe space, you're able to share your emotions freely. This helps you to process and regulate them in a healthy way, leading to positive outcomes. Opening up to a trusted family member or a friend can offer you the emotional rest you need.

While this might seem scary at first, it's essential to express your feelings – including any uncomfortable ones – to lighten the burden; otherwise, you risk compromising your mental well-being.

Emotional rest is also about identifying people and situations you find draining. Make a list of what drains you and, if possible, engage less with the things on this list. Another way to seek emotional rest is to keep a journal, as this will help you express any feelings you may have bottled up.

Everyone goes through bumpy times, but if you're feeling low for days, seek professional advice.

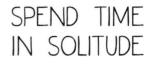

# SPEND TIME IN SOLITUDE

Choosing to spend time alone is not the same as feeling lonely. Loneliness is when you're disconnected from people, while solitude is a free, fulfilling, warm space away from chaos, where you can be yourself. Research shows that introverts are more enthusiastic about solitude, but everyone can benefit from alone time.

In fact, solitude is a proven stress reducer and confidence-booster – it nurtures your sense of self, helps you gather your thoughts and feelings and allows you to discover new insights about yourself. It can also spark creative ideas.

Let solitude recharge your batteries. Why not take yourself off alone for a coffee or to browse books in a library?

Within you,
there is a stillness
and a sanctuary to
which you can retreat
at any time and
be yourself.

**HERMANN
HESSE**

# Take micro-breaks

The human body is built to thrive by being active in a series of short sprints. This is why taking a break, even for a few minutes, can offer you the refresh you need in your day. Take a micro-break of 1 to 2 minutes every hour. Try these activities:

- Roll your shoulders gently.

- Make a cup of tea mindfully. Notice the aromas, the sound of the kettle boiling, the heat coming from the mug.

- Drink your tea slowly. Notice the flavours and sensations in your mouth.

- Gaze out of the window.

- Stretch your legs, wriggle your toes.

- Listen to music.

- Take deep breaths for 1 minute.

- Watch a short funny video clip.

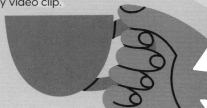

# TUNE IN TO PAUSES

In today's online world we're accessible to everyone all the time, which leaves many of us stressed or worn out. If you're constantly bombarded by work emails or messages, tune in to longer pauses to calm your body's fight-or-flight response (how you react to danger or stress) and prevent burnout.

A simple break like an afternoon off or enjoying a film might be the perfect tonic. But if you're completely drained then you need deeper, good quality rest, such as getting enough sleep and allowing yourself to really relax. If you can, consider taking a longer break such as a weekend away or a holiday.

Remember to prioritize relaxation and set clear boundaries between your downtime and other demands.

# T REFLECTING

Rest and reflection go hand in hand. When the outside world becomes our central focus, it's easy to forget to look inward. Taking the time to stop and reflect is not only an important skill, it also renews your perspective on what matters to you the most, what you're grateful for and how you wish to spend your time, and it helps you to celebrate all you have learned.

If we know what's going on within ourselves, we stand a better chance of navigating the world around us. Think of some questions to ask yourself daily, weekly or monthly and write them in your journal.

Try asking yourself how you feel today, what you achieved this week or what you could improve on. Reflection will help you become better in every way because learning to embrace yourself will boost your confidence and restore your sense of self.

Try reflecting during these everyday restful activities:

- Take a 30-minute walk in nature.

- Listen to your thoughts and feelings.

- When feeling a little stressed, set a timer for 5 minutes to write down your thoughts.

# DO NOTHING

Every now and then it's important to do absolutely nothing. You don't always need to be getting things done and some days it's perfectly okay to be unproductive, especially when you're worn out.

If you're feeling overstretched and weary, give yourself permission to say no and achieve nothing in particular. Slow down, breathe and simply be. Take time to decompress.

We all need times of inactivity to rest and recover. You're not weak for doing nothing and you're certainly not lazy – sometimes it's the most productive and nourishing thing you can do.

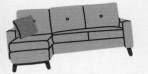

# STOP THE BUSYNESS

When you're consumed by a hectic lifestyle, your mental health is at risk. There's no denying that busyness causes a huge amount of stress and anxiety, and this mental overwhelm can affect anyone.

What makes rest so difficult is that many people feel guilty about taking time for themselves. You might feel that by resting you're being indulgent or wasting time, while busyness can sometimes be mistaken for a sign of status – making you feel important or valued. But this is harmful to your well-being. To escape the busyness of life, you need to pause and breathe. Not everything is about accomplishments and work tasks. Your health and happiness matter. Remember, it's necessary to rest, so don't feel bad about doing it.

# REAL REST
# FEELS LIKE
# EVERY CELL IS
## THANKING YOU
## FOR TAKING
## CARE OF YOU.

JENNIFER WILLIAMSON

# Rest Your Mind

Most of us spend a lot of time stuck in our minds. We might be preoccupied with the past, worrying about the future or simply trying to get through our to-do lists. But spending too much time engaging with unhelpful thoughts can have a detrimental effect on our mental health and self-esteem. In fact, science tells us that we're on autopilot nearly half our lives – no wonder we're so exhausted! This is where the power of resting your mind comes in. Here's how to do just that...

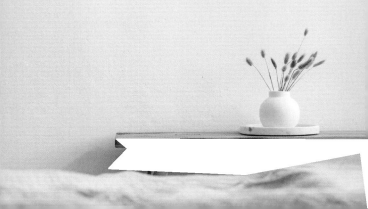

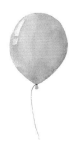

# LET YOUR WORRIES GO

We all worry from time to time, but when unhelpful thoughts start to spiral out of control, they can overwhelm us. This is why it's helpful to stop them in their tracks. Often the act of physically releasing worries can help them go away. Grab a piece of paper and write down your top three bothersome thoughts. Then rip the paper into little pieces and throw it in the recycle bin. Or try visualizing some balloons with your worries trapped inside. Close your eyes and imagine them floating away. Hopefully they'll take some of your stress with them!

YOU ARE TODAY
WHERE YOUR
THOUGHTS HAVE
BROUGHT YOU;
YOU WILL BE
TOMORROW
WHERE YOUR
THOUGHTS
TAKE YOU.

*James Allen*

# AND BREATHE...

Life can be bumpy, but that doesn't mean you can't handle it. One way to help is meditation. Studies show this ancient practice offers many benefits, including helping to relieve depression, anxiety and chronic pain.

When we are tense, our breathing is in our upper chest, but when we breathe meditatively we are actively focusing on our breath, drawing it deep into our belly. Paying attention to our breath grounds us in the present moment and calms unhelpful thoughts.

## Breathing meditation

Put all distractions away and take time to be still. Find a comfortable place to sit. Play soothing music or nature sounds if you wish. Set a timer for 5 to 10 minutes. Gently close your eyes and notice your breathing. Notice the inhalation and the exhalation. Pay attention to how the air feels when it enters your lungs. Take a deep breath in through your nose, fill your lungs, then exhale through your mouth and repeat.

Keep focusing on your breathing as best you can. If your mind wanders, that's okay, simply guide it back to your breathing. When the timer is up, gently open your eyes. Notice how you feel.

Bear in mind there are many types of meditation, from focusing on the breath to guided meditations, so keep trying them until you find one that works for you.

# Get colouring

Try switching off your thinking mind by spending time doing something creative, like drawing or colouring. Just choose an activity that doesn't cause you stress, as the aim is to quieten your pesky thoughts and give your brain a much-needed break.

Try using a colouring book for 10 minutes daily. Start by sitting still, with a straight posture, and notice your breathing; then begin to colour. To be even more mindful, use cool colours rather than bright ones, as doing so is confidence boosting and brings a sense of calm.

If you don't have a colouring book, print an online design or draw your own.

# THE POWER OF NO

If there are tasks or events coming up which will overstretch you, stress you out or won't make you happy, put yourself first and say no. This could be declining a work project that isn't right for you or an invitation to go out. Putting yourself first is an act of self-care that sets the tone for how you would like to be treated, so when you look after yourself, your relationships improve too.

Give yourself permission to say no. Go at your pace, do whatever makes your soul happy – it's not your job to please everyone.

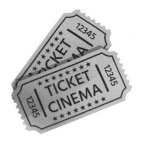

# ESCAPE WITH A FILM

When you're tired, flopping in front of the TV and immersing yourself in an easy-watching film can be hugely restorative. In fact, it's backed up by science – escapist viewing helps people cope when they're feeling anxious, because while you're watching something, there isn't an expectation to keep conversation flowing. Even better, put on a comedy. Laughter has been shown to decrease stress hormones and release feel-good endorphins which help you to relax. So treat yourself to a movie night with your favourite snacks and a cosy blanket, and escape for a little while.

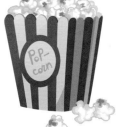

# CENTRE YOURSELF

Mandalas (Sanskrit for "circle" or "centre") are circular designs that have repeating patterns and colours radiating from the centre. Creating mandalas is a form of therapy which refreshes the brain, boosts the immune system, lessens anxiety and induces relaxation by calming the nervous system.

Beyond their vibrant appearance, mandalas hold an even deeper meaning in Hindu and Buddhist philosophy, which teach that moving toward the centre transforms suffering into joy. Drawing or colouring circles can help bring us back to our own centre by offering stability to a wobbly mind.

Download free mandalas online or use colouring apps to start centring yourself today.

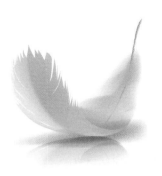

# PASSION
# IS ENERGY.
FEEL THE POWER
THAT COMES FROM
FOCUSING ON WHAT
EXCITES YOU.

**OPRAH WINFREY**

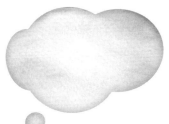

# Take time to daydream

Where did your mind wander off to during your last meeting? Perhaps you were thinking about what to eat for dinner or your last beach holiday. Daydreaming can be an instant mood-lifter and, when done in moderation, it's been shown to help manage anxiety, spark creativity and strengthen relationships.

Research shows that many of us spend up to 6 hours a day staring at screens. It's no surprise the mind resists boredom when there's so much stimulation. Try to find time in your day to allow your mind to be bored. Let it wander instead of listening to music or podcasts on your commute or while loading the dishwasher.

# THE POWER OF WALKING

Walking is powerful. By simply slowing your pace down you can refresh and renew your perspective on the chaos of the world and your thoughts. Sometimes when you're strolling, answers to problems unfold as you clear your head. Research shows it's a great way to tap into creativity – in fact, walking for 5 minutes every hour for 6 hours helps you feel rested and improves fitness levels.

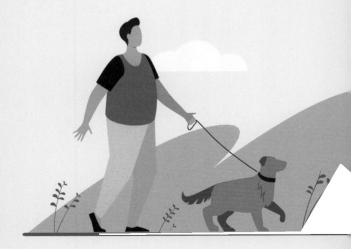

If you don't feel motivated to go for a walk, think of it as going for a rest. Here's how to try mindful walking:

- Start by slowing your pace. Pay attention to each step – notice the sensations in the soles of your feet. Then notice clouds floating, the colour of the sky. Now listen to birdsongs, breathe in the aromas of freshly cut grass or flowers in bloom. If you pick up a drink along the way, pay attention to the flavours and temperature.

- Research shows that walking in the great outdoors has a lasting impact on your mental health, leaving you feeling happier all day. It doesn't have to be a long hike in exotic nature; simply being outside is enough. So pull on your comfy shoes and step outside to clear your mind.

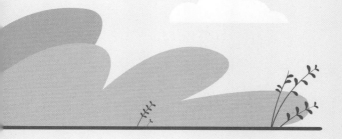

# Become a bookworm

Reading for pleasure is restful and enriches you in many ways. By using time more wisely, you could add years to your life: studies show a daily 30-minute reading session can help you live two years longer. Not only does reading enhance emotional intelligence and empathy, but it can also reduce stress levels by up to 68 per cent, as well as slow your heart rate and soothe muscle tension.

Wake up 30 minutes earlier to read a book in bed, or sit on a park bench to get the benefits of being in nature too.

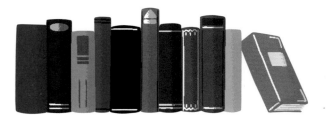

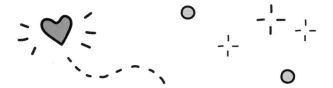

# GET DOODLING

Have you ever scribbled patterns or shapes while your attention is elsewhere? Doodling freely is not only fun, it also helps you to concentrate, express feelings and lower stress by allowing the brain to find lost fragments of memories and bring them to the present. As you then start filling in these missing gaps, doodling can help you feel more relaxed by making sense of your life.

To get started, draw repetitive squares, circles, lines or spirals. Doodle for 5 minutes daily – you don't have to be Van Gogh! Add your doodles to your journal entries to help big-picture thinking.

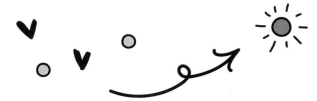

# RETREAT AND REPLENISH

While your social media feed might be full of people indulging in tropical retreats where they spend their days sipping juice, detoxing and attending yoga classes, it might not be a practical option for you.

But don't let that stop you. It's possible to create a retreat in the comfort of your own home.

Choose a suitable time and let people know you're unavailable then. Switch off all distractions or lock them away if you don't have the willpower to resist checking.

Ensure you have your favourite food, drink, music, candles, books, colouring or whatever relaxation items you choose. You could even keep these in a box for when you want to retreat.

Next, choose the place you will retreat to – does it need tidying, warming or cooling? Should it be vibrant, calming or comforting? Bring in whatever creates this ambience. Pick comfortable clothes and enough layers to keep warm.

Begin by lighting a candle or reading inspirational quotes. This is your time to be still, write, paint and do as you wish without interruption.

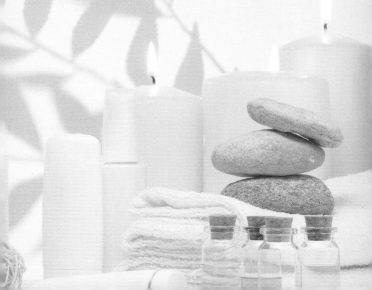

Music gives
a soul to the universe,
wings to the mind,
flight to the imagination
and life to everything.

PLATO

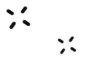

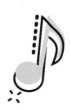

# TUNE IN TO THE BEAT

When you're feeling miserable, there's always that one song which turns the corners of your mouth up, lifting your spirit. Music relaxes you, connects you to your emotions and distracts you from worrying thoughts.

Play a song you love. Really listen to the music. Pay attention to how the beats connect with your body. Notice how the lyrics resonate with your feelings. What instruments can you pick out? Focus on the music and let your thoughts fade away. You could sing along and dance, or just close your eyes and unwind.

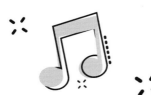

# FIVE-MINUTE MIND-BOOSTERS

Even with just a few spare minutes, you can give your mind a yearned-for rest. Here's how:

- Start your day with a mindful shower. Instead of focusing on your to-do list, notice the fragrance of the soap, the sensation and temperature of the water trickling through your fingers.

- Get outside with a cup of tea and catch the sun rising. Notice the colours and birdsong.

- Sip a glass of water slowly. Pay attention to how you feel. Keep well hydrated because dehydration leads to higher levels of the stress hormone cortisol.

- If you've been in back-to-back online meetings, get up, move your body, release any tension and sit in a different place to renew your perspective.

- Lighting a candle can instantly stimulate relaxing vibes and give your mind a little rest. Use calming scents such as lavender or citrus and watch the flame flicker for a few minutes, noticing the shapes, colours and aromas.

- When a wave of worry or anxious thoughts kicks in, rest your head between your knees, below your heart, and take deep, slow breaths for an immediate calming effect.

# PUZZLE AND CHILL

How satisfying does it feel when you complete a puzzle? When your hard work and patience pay off, you get a sense of accomplishment. Research shows puzzling helps to ease stress and anxiety, slows memory loss and delays the onset of dementia. When you are focusing your attention on a problem that needs to be solved, whether that's finding a pattern in numbers or searching for a matching edge, your mind switches off from the problems you've been dwelling on, leaving you feeling calmer.

As well as puzzling alone, why not try it on a date night, as part of a team-building day or on family holidays? A shared challenge is a fabulous, relaxing way to strengthen bonds with people.

# Dream holiday

If you can't get away on holiday, use your imagination to transport yourself to a delightfully serene place. Recall somewhere you found relaxing or think of a sanctuary you'd like to visit.

Gently close your eyes. Let your imagination transport you there. What sounds, shapes, colours, tastes, aromas, temperatures can you conjure up? You might imagine a warm beach, sounds of gentle waves crashing, the smell of tropical flowers, the taste of cool vanilla ice cream. Relax in this dreamy place for a little while.

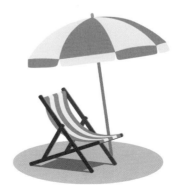

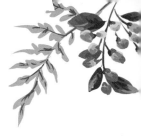
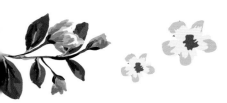

# TAKE TIME
# FOR YOURSELF

No matter how busy your schedule is, take time for yourself every single day. Even if it's just 5 to 10 minutes to sit and relax or try a tip from this book, prioritize putting rest first. You can even schedule time to rest – set reminders if you need to.

By taking time for yourself, you will feel happier and more in control because you'll be able to put the demands of life into perspective. You'll also have the opportunity to check in with yourself and see if your needs are being met, which is especially helpful if you're feeling tired and out of sorts.

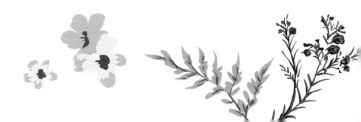

# ALMOST EVERYTHING WILL WORK AGAIN IF YOU UNPLUG IT FOR A FEW MINUTES,

INCLUDING YOU.

**ANNE LAMOTT**

# Rest Your Body

Life is exhausting. Whether you're commuting to work, caring for your family or trying to squeeze in exercise, hobbies and meeting up with friends, it's no surprise you barely have time to stop and truly recharge your body. But it's so important to take time to give your physical self all the comfort and nourishment you need, because when you do, you'll be recharged and stronger, and ready to live your best life.

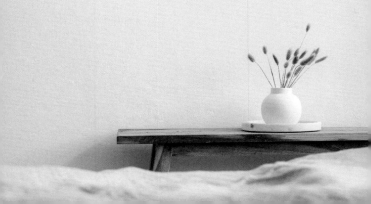

# BATHING RITUAL

Since ancient times, immersing our bodies in water has been known for its healing benefits. Some studies have shown that even the sight or sound of water can trigger a flood of neurochemicals that promote relaxation and increase blood flow to the heart and brain.

Try your own bathing ritual. Light scented candles, play relaxing music, infuse warm water with bath salts or your favourite oils (try lavender or chamomile) – this will all help rejuvenate your muscles and leave you feeling serene. Undress mindfully: imagine stripping away any negativity with your clothes. Slide into the warm water, then breathe, rest and relax – you deserve it.

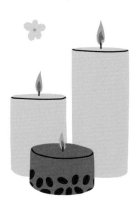

KEEP YOUR
EYES ON
THE STARS,
AND YOUR
FEET ON THE
GROUND.

*Theodore Roosevelt*

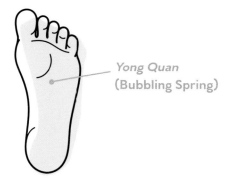

*Yong Quan*
(Bubbling Spring)

# TREAT YOUR FEET

We use our feet a lot throughout the day – walking, standing, exercising, getting 10,000 steps in. There's no doubt they're putting in long hours, often without the care and attention they deserve. Interestingly, there are many invigorating acupressure points on the soles of our feet which calm restlessness and improve circulation. Massage your soles or stand in the sunshine, bare feet on the ground, and breathe deeply to release tension. For an instant refresh, apply pressure to the special point known as *Yong Quan* (Bubbling Spring). If you have more time, add approximately 100 g Epsom salts to a large bowl of warm water and soak your feet for up to 30 minutes to soothe away soreness.

# Scan your body

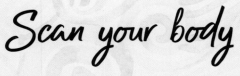

When you're stressed, your nervous system reacts, which raises your blood pressure and levels of the stress hormones adrenaline and cortisol, leaving you feeling out of sorts. Breathing from your belly disrupts this stress response and takes your body back to a restful state.

Try this simple body scan to release stored tension and get in touch with your physical self.

Sitting comfortably, place your hands on your thighs. Close your eyes and focus on your breathing. Notice the presence of your body.

Now, pay attention to your head, forehead and eyes – invite them to soften and relax. Next, notice your neck and shoulders – allow them to drop and loosen. Scan your entire body, noticing your upper back, chest, belly, lower back, pelvis, legs and feet. Pay attention to any numbness, aches, tingling, tightness and whether your body feels hot or cold. Breathe deeply, wriggle your fingers and toes, and gently open your eyes. Observe how you feel afterward.

# GET ACTIVE

Getting active might seem a contradictory way to rest, but some studies have shown that repetitive movements, such as running, have a meditative effect on the brain. This is because while your mind is focused on the physical task at hand, your chattering brain is resting.

Exercise itself, even strenuous activities like weightlifting or cycling, can be restful if you love it, providing you rest afterward. Try mindful swimming or paddleboarding. Instead of listening to bothersome thoughts, tune in to your breathing. Notice your heart rate, the temperature of the water and any sensations in the soles of your feet during exercise.

# REST YOUR HANDS

We often take our hands for granted, but they do so much for us: brushing our teeth, grasping keys, turning doorknobs, zipping our clothes, making cups of tea, typing messages, lighting candles, turning pages, baking cakes, picking flowers, hugging people – the list is endless.

Pay attention to your hands today. Massage the bones of your hands and the webbing between your fingers using your index finger and thumb. For each finger and thumb, think of a reason you're grateful for your hands. By taking breaks to care for your hands, you'll prevent aches and strains.

# Playtime

Play is important for your happiness and health, which is no surprise as laughter instantly relaxes your muscles and lifts your mood. As you grow older and the responsibilities of adulthood weigh you down, you often lose the freedom to enjoy fun activities you once loved. What do you miss doing? Perhaps it's lying in a hammock, rolling down a grassy hill or sitting on a swing. Choose one exciting thing to do today and see how it makes you feel.

You can enjoy fun activities with friends and family, rekindle an old hobby or perhaps even try a new one, as long as it doesn't add any extra pressure.

*Balance in the body is the foundation for balance in life.*

B. K. S. IYENGAR

# STRETCH YOUR BODY

You don't have to be super bendy or ultra-fit to try yoga. Research shows yoga relaxes your entire body and nervous system, improves circulation and strengthens the mind—body connection. For an instant reset, try the following poses.

## Mountain Pose
Stand with your feet hip distance apart and your arms by your side, palms face up. Lengthen your tail bone toward the floor and tighten your thighs, drawing your shoulder blades down and together. Soften your gaze and breathe deeply. Hold for at least 30 seconds.

## Child's Pose
Kneel with your feet together, toes tucked under and your knees wide. Lower your bottom toward your feet, stretching your upper body forward and down with your arms extended.

# MAKE A MEAL OF IT

Mealtimes can be restorative – even the humblest meal will nourish your soul if you slow down a little. Many of us eat on the go and often miss out on really tasting our food. Here's how to make mealtimes a mindful, restful daily ritual:

- Pour love and attention into your meals by concentrating on chopping and stirring, noticing scents, textures and colours.

- Reframe cooking to see it as rest time rather than a chore.

- Make mealtimes special: set your table with care; place a small jar of flowers or candles as a centrepiece; use enticing presentation, for example a sprinkling of fresh herbs; put screens away.

- Eat slowly, noticing flavours, fragrances, textures.

# LISTEN TO YOUR GUT

Our digestive system plays a hugely important role in keeping nutrients flowing to essential organs and systems. During hectic or stressful times, it's easy to eat on the go, overeat or skip meals altogether. Many convenience foods are laden with hidden salts, sugars and pollutants, which puts a strain on our digestive system and can lead to bloating, discomfort or lethargy. Thankfully, with a few simple changes you can reboot your digestive system to be more efficient and give you that feel-good energy boost you need. Try the following:

- Cut down your alcohol intake. If you want to drink socially, try diluting your drink with water or swapping every other alcoholic drink for a soft one.

- Reduce tea or coffee intake gradually by a cup a day. Replace with caffeine-free herbal drinks such as peppermint or ginger, or honey and lemon for an energy uplift.

- If you smoke, consider beginning your journey toward quitting.

- Cleanse your diet by limiting sugary and processed foods. Pick fresh food and ingredients whenever possible.

- Drink plenty of water throughout the day to clear toxins. Fill a clear bottle of water to keep with you and monitor your intake.

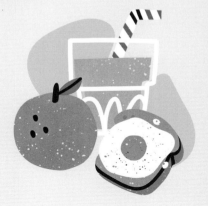

# CONNECT WITH NATURE

Connecting with nature can boost your physical and mental health. Few of us spend time in nature in a really mindful way, but it doesn't have to be like this. Follow these simple techniques to connect with nature:

- Go to a park, garden or, even better, a wild place. First, simply sit on the ground allowing your body to connect with the earth. Close your eyes and get curious, allowing your senses to tune in to the soundscape around you – the far-off birdsong and tinier sounds of insects nearby. You'll be amazed by what you hear if you really listen. Spend at least 15 minutes doing so.

- On a walk, focus on nature's gifts, such as leaves, stones, flower petals, grass blades, feathers and sticks. Observe as if it's the first time you're seeing nature: pick things up, notice textures or colours (but please don't pick wild flowers).

- Have a go at the Japanese practice of forest bathing. Find a quiet spot in a forest or among trees and try to leave all distractions behind. Stand or sit and use your senses to soak up fresh oxygen, the pleasing colours and textures of bark, wind rustling through branches and the breeze on your face.

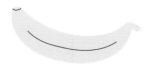

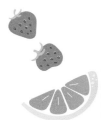

# JUICE BOOST

Fruit and vegetables are uplifting, soothing and nutrient-rich, and help your body to heal. Try these nurturing drinks for an instant body boost:

### Build-me-up juice

Root vegetables revitalize the blood by enhancing circulation and oxygen levels, promoting good gut health and lifting your energy levels. Juice 1 carrot, 1 beetroot, 2 celery sticks, a 1 cm (2 ½ in.) piece of ginger and ½ a lemon, then top up with coconut water.

### Pick-me-up juice

Antioxidant-rich berries help to improve your energy levels and immunity. Blend a handful of raspberries, blackberries, blueberries and a pinch of cinnamon, then add coconut water to the desired thickness.

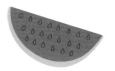
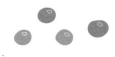

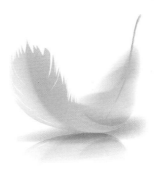

**SOMETIMES
LETTING THINGS
GO IS AN ACT
OF FAR GREATER
POWER**
THAN DEFENDING
OR HANGING ON.

ECKHART TOLLE

# RELAX YOUR MUSCLES

We all feel stressed sometimes and it's normal to hold that tension in our muscles without realizing. Progressive muscle relaxation is an effective therapy that helps you to release tension by deliberately tightening and then relaxing your muscles one at a time. Studies show it can help sleep problems, anxiety and high blood pressure. Try this:

- Sit or lie comfortably, close your eyes. Take five slow deep breaths. Starting at your toes, tense your muscles, hold for a count of three then release.

- Tense all the major muscle groups from your toes and fingers to your shoulders, neck and facial muscles. Then relax them. Notice how you feel afterward.

# Self-soothing head massage

Most people love having their scalp massaged as it helps to switch off for a little while. Along with instant relaxation, a head massage can promote healthy hair, relieve headaches and lower stress. Try these simple steps to give yourself a soothing head massage:

- Sit comfortably, close your eyes and allow yourself to relax.

- Using the fingers and thumbs of both hands, apply firm pressure to your head with your fingertips and move them in small circular motions. Use oils such as sweet almond or peppermint for extra nourishment.

- Massage your entire head before moving down the sides of your neck and along your shoulders to release tension.

# LEARN TO BREATHE

Most of us take breathing for granted, but we breathe too shallowly, using only a tiny portion of our lungs. Breathing properly is vital for supplying oxygen to organs, calming nerves, normalizing blood pressure, improving sleep and regulating our metabolism as well as helping to heal numerous medical conditions.

Luckily, learning how to breathe using simple exercises will bring truly marvellous benefits for your mind and body. Try this yogic breathing:

- Sit comfortably. Lengthen your spine. Relax your shoulders. Close your eyes and mouth.

- Rest your hands on your belly. Inhale deeply through your nose, drawing the breath into your belly. Notice your belly expanding. Exhale slowly through your nose. Feel your belly contract. Repeat two more times.

- On your next breath, inhale to a count of five, exhaling slowly for ten counts. Notice your belly contract. Repeat five more times: inhaling for five, exhaling for ten.

- Upon finishing, let your breathing return to its natural rate. Feel the soothing, wholesome energy flowing through your body.

- Practise this exercise daily and at any time you feel overwhelmed in order to establish healthy breathing patterns. You can also try online breathing tutorials, but speak to your doctor first if you have any medical conditions that affect your breathing.

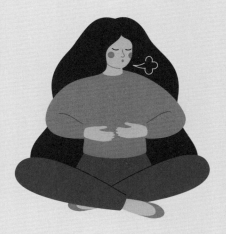

# CREATE A HOME SPA

A little pampering goes a long way, especially when you're exhausted. The tranquillity that comes with the fresh candles and scented oils as soon as you step into a spa is truly relaxing – and there's nothing stopping you from creating your own spa experience at home.

To create relaxing spa vibes, scatter petals in a warm bath along with drops of your favourite essential oil, then light a candle and play soothing sounds. Curate your own spa menu or use this book for ideas: you could try a bathing ritual (page 57), treat your feet (page 59), rest your hands (page 63) and finish with a body-boosting juice (page 72).

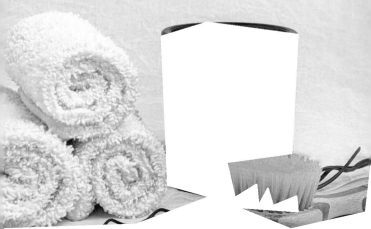

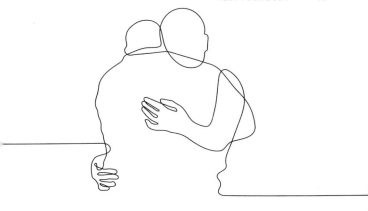

# EMBRACE LIFE

Hugging is often comforting because it releases the hormone oxytocin, which promotes trust and empathy while also triggering our anti-stress response and leaving us feeling relaxed and safe. Hugs are also proven to boost energy and they are not just limited to an embrace with people. Stroking or even just making eye contact with a pet can release oxytocin, while hugging trees has been shown to activate this feel-good hormone too. Find someone or something to hug and, as you wrap your arms around your chosen person, animal or tree, feel your body release the tension it's been carrying.

# IT ALWAYS PAYS TO DWELL SLOWLY ON THE BEAUTIFUL THINGS –

## THE MORE BEAUTIFUL THE MORE SLOWLY

ATTICUS

# Welcome to Sleep

Good sleep is essential for our health and happiness. Everything seems so much brighter after a good night's shut-eye and most of us wish we had more. When your sleep is broken, you're likely to feel drowsy or forgetful and nothing seems right. Sleep issues affect 45 per cent of the world's population, which is hardly surprising when so many of us are bogged down by to-do lists and constantly bombarded with stimuli. Good quality sleep helps your body to recover and allows you to wake up refreshed. Read on to tune in to the power of sleep.

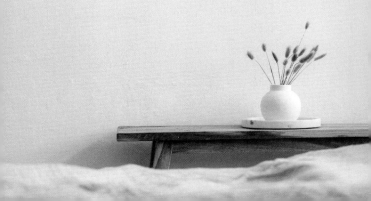

# WHY YOU NEED SLEEP

Sleep is a basic human need. We spend up to one-third of our lives sleeping and studies suggest that a lack of sleep damages immune system function, prevents our nervous system from working properly and can lead to drowsiness, broken memory and impaired daily performance as well as health problems such as obesity, diabetes, anxiety and depression.

Sleep gives our cells the chance to repair from daily activity and helps our decision-making, social interactions and emotional functioning. It also maintains optimum release of hormones, particularly the growth hormone.

# GOOD SLEEP, GOOD HEALTH

Good-quality sleep can do so much for you. When your body gets the sleep it needs, your immune system also gets the rest it needs to boost your immunity and fight off pathogens such as colds and other viruses.

Studies show sleep helps prevent weight gain and improves memory, processing and consolidating your memories from the day. Sleep also boosts your heart health by reducing cortisol levels, the presence of which makes your heart work harder, and allowing your heart the rest it needs to function healthily. Of course, sleep also boosts your daily mood and performance.

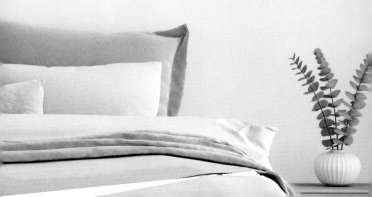

# What is sleep?

Sleep allows your brain and body to slow down and engage in recovery processes. Disrupting these complex processes has a negative impact on your well-being.

During sleep, you go through four to five sleep cycles and each cycle consists of four distinct sleep stages. These four stages are broken down further into rapid eye movement (REM) sleep and non-REM (NREM) sleep – both are important and have very different functions.

Stages one to three are NREM sleep, which enables restoration in the form of building muscles, regenerating cells and strengthening your immune system.

Stage one is short – dozing off to sleep. Stage two is when your body and mind slow down while you fall asleep. It's easy to be woken during these stages. Deep sleep happens during stage three, when brain activity slows and your body rests further into recovery and healing.

Stage four is REM sleep, when brain activity increases to similar levels to when you're awake, which is why this stage is linked to intense dreams. Curiously, our heart rate and breathing elevate during this stage but most muscles are inactive, preventing us from playing out those dreams. Each sleep cycle lasts between 70 and 120 minutes.

IT IS HEALTH
THAT IS REAL
WEALTH
AND NOT
PIECES OF
GOLD AND
SILVER.

*Mahatma Gandhi*

# KNOW YOUR BODY CLOCK

The sleep–wake cycle is an example of a circadian rhythm. Your body has an internal clock which regulates vital functions. The circadian rhythm is a 24-hour cycle that influences alertness, hunger, metabolism, fertility and mood and is synchronized with the main body clock in the brain.

Daylight triggers your main body clock to send signals to keep you alert. As darkness falls, the main clock starts producing melatonin, a sleep-promoting hormone. It sends signals throughout the night to keep you asleep. Your circadian rhythm establishes your sleep–wake cycle with day and night, and when thrown off balance it leads to sleep problems and insomnia.

# GET ENOUGH SLEEP

Most of us need between 7 and 9 hours of shut-eye every night. Teenagers and children need a lot more. Factors such as work demands, daily niggles, health and sleeping environment can stop you from getting enough sleep. Of course, healthy lifestyle habits can positively impact sleep quality.

But sometimes people get so used to sleep deprivation that it becomes normalized and they run on empty even though their brains and bodies struggle. This can lead to a higher risk of conditions such as obesity, diabetes, heart disease, high blood pressure, poor mental health and even to premature death.

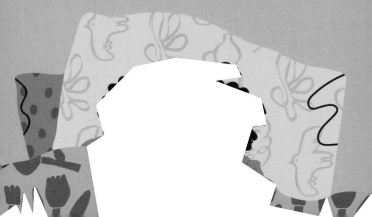

# SLEEP FACTS

- Jet lag is worse when you fly eastward because your circadian cycle is slightly longer than 24 hours (it gets worse the more time zones you cross).

- People with severe insomnia are seven times more likely to have work-related accidents than good sleepers are.

- A study shows 78 per cent of people are more excited to go to bed if they have fresh-smelling sheets.

- Across a large population of sleepers, approximately 54 per cent of time in bed was spent sleeping on their side, 38 per cent sleeping on their back and 7 per cent sleeping on their stomach.

- Premenstrual syndrome makes women at least two times as likely to report insomnia-like symptoms.

# SWEET DREAMS

We all dream, whether or not we remember it in the morning. Our dreams can be in the first person, involuntary and illogical; they can involve people and trigger strong emotions, and they may include parts of our waking life.

Science tells us dreaming may help to build memory, process emotions and assist the brain to purge unnecessary information. But dreams can sometimes help you figure out a problem that has been troubling you while you've been awake. Whether they are pleasant or disturbing, your dreams might show you a different way of tackling the problems you're facing in your daily life.

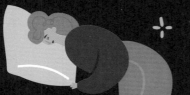

So, explore your dreams with curiosity. To capture them, say your dream out loud or tell someone about it. You might like to write or draw in your journal – doing so can help you understand your dreams or see if there is anything that might help you work out your real-life troubles. Think about who you see in your dreams, look for shapes and symbols, hear the sounds or smell the fragrances. Sometimes rituals and affirmations before bedtime can lead to pleasant dreams.

Why not treat yourself to a gorgeous uplifting journal to keep by your bedside to record your dreams immediately upon rising?

A good laugh
and a long sleep
are the best cures in
the doctor's book.

**IRISH PROVERB**

# FACE YOUR NIGHTMARES

It's entirely normal for unpleasant dreams to feel a little disturbing or even wake us, but they're not truly threatening. Some people believe nightmares can convey messages and that anxiety can influence dreams: for example, using the toilet in public can symbolize having no outlet for self-expression; being naked, a fear of showing your true self; public speaking, a fear of getting it wrong. But of course this isn't always the case.

It can be helpful to acknowledge unpleasant dreams. You don't have to dwell on them; simply jot down what your subconscious mind is telling you. If frequent nightmares disturb your sleep, speak with your doctor or therapist to help lessen worries.

# SLEEP AND MENTAL HEALTH

We often take sleep for granted, but it's important to note that sleep and mental health are intertwined. Mental health disorders can make it harder to sleep well, while poor-quality sleep can trigger or worsen mental health difficulties. Lack of sleep has been linked to depression and has been shown to worsen the symptoms of many other conditions, including depression, anxiety and bipolar disorder.

Of course, sleep and mental health are complex and affect people in individual ways, but research has suggested that improving sleep can have a positive impact on mental health – sleep is incorporated in treatments for some psychiatric disorders.

Often sleep problems are caused by insufficient self-care around sleep. The chapters "Sleep Self-Care" and "Good Nights" show you how to promote better sleep.

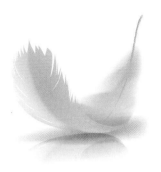

**HAPPINESS
CONSISTS
OF GETTING
ENOUGH SLEEP.**
JUST THAT,
NOTHING MORE.

ROBERT A. HEINLEIN

# More sleep, fewer low moods

Imagine sleep as music. When you sleep well, the music is uplifting and positive – you face life with optimism and people are lovely. After a terrible night's sleep, the tone of the music sounds heavy, everything seems gloomy and people and events are seen through a negative lens. You're likely to feel grumpy, to overreact and feel less excited when good things happen because the prefrontal cortex (the part of the brain that helps us regulate emotions) is muted.

Studies show even partially sleep-deprived people report an increase in negative moods, such as frustration, irritability, anger and sadness, and far fewer positive moods.

Although we might be tempted to stay up late to meet those deadlines or finish that episode on Netflix, deep sleep is so important because it soothes the body's fight-or-flight response and gives us important neurochemicals such as dopamine (the reward chemical) and norepinephrine (which contributes to the fight-or-flight response), which recharge us with positive energy.

Lack of sleep is particularly harmful to consolidating positive emotional memories and is closely linked with mood disorders. This means ongoing sleeplessness lowers your mood and increases negative day-to-day experiences, but your mood also affects how well you sleep. Read on for tips on how to get better sleep and lift your mood.

# TOO MUCH SLEEP

You need 7 to 9 hours of sleep for optimum functioning, although sleeping too much can have a detrimental impact on you too. People with hypersomnia (sleeping too much) feel overly sleepy during the day and might struggle to stay awake when needed. Studies suggest hypersomnia is linked with reduced deep sleep and an increase in NREM sleep.

If you're napping often during the day and still have low energy, sleep for long hours at night, fall asleep while talking or have difficulty remembering things, try the tips in the chapters "Sleep Self-Care" and "Good Nights". If symptoms persist, speak with your doctor.

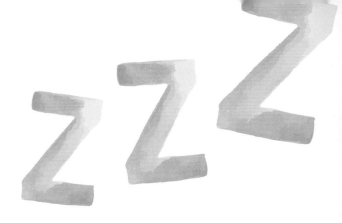

# SNORING

We all snore from time to time: snoring affects 40 per cent of women and 57 per cent of men. Snoring happens during deep sleep when our muscles loosen and the airway at the back of our throat narrows and vibrates, causing tissues to make rattling sounds as we breathe in and out.

Occasional snoring is normal and is easily helped with lifestyle changes such as losing weight if you're overweight, sleeping on your side, avoiding smoking, not drinking too much alcohol and cutting out sleeping pills, which can trigger snoring. Sometimes snoring is caused by a health condition, so consider getting help if necessary (see page 104).

# DOZING FUN FACTS

- Humans are the only mammals that voluntarily put off sleeping until later. Imagine how wonderful it must be to sleep anytime, anywhere.

- Sleeping on your front can help digestion, while lying on your left side helps to lessen heartburn.

- The record for the longest duration without sleep is 11 days – achieved in 1964 by American student Randy Gardner. This is absolutely not recommended!

# Unplug and recharge

Too much time spent on screens is linked with poor sleep quality, high cortisol levels and anxiety. It can be hard to unplug from screens: they're often in such close proximity it's no wonder we feel compelled to check them when notifications are blinking away.

Create little pockets of screen-free time during the day to recharge. Set some boundaries, such as no phones during mealtimes or while you have company. Try putting your phone on silent for an hour or so to avoid constant distractions, or perhaps delete some apps or mute a group chat so you don't feel pressurized to respond immediately.

# INSOMNIA

It's worrying and horrible when you can't fall asleep: you're lying in bed wide awake in desperate need of recharging your batteries to face the busy day ahead. You finally doze off but you're tossing and turning throughout the night and wake ridiculously early, which leaves you feeling groggy, irritable and with little energy to focus. You struggle to keep your eyes open throughout the day and by 3 p.m. you're yawning. This is insomnia – it throws your sleep and circadian rhythm off balance, leaving you without enough proper rest. Insomnia is believed to affect approximately 33 per cent of the world's population.

Often, insomnia is caused by stresses of life such as work pressures, money worries and concerns about health or family. Traumatic events, such as the death or illness of a loved one, divorce or job loss, can play a role in insomnia.

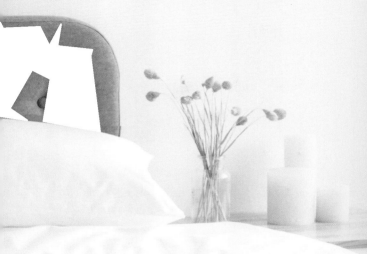

Sometimes travel or shift work may disrupt your circadian rhythms, or you might have poor sleep self-care, such as irregular bedtimes, eating meals too late, an uncomfortable sleeping environment or not unwinding in the evening, especially away from screens.

Thankfully, many of these factors can be addressed using the tips in this book, but if insomnia is making it hard for you to function, speak with your doctor.

# KNOW WHEN TO GET HELP

As you have seen, sleep is an incredibly complex process which is influenced by many different factors. While there are plenty of lifestyle and practical tips in this book to promote better-quality sleep, there are also a number of sleep disorders that need professional medical diagnosis and treatment.

It is important to become aware of your sleep, so think about keeping a record of your sleeping patterns in a journal. If you notice that you're suffering from persistent symptoms or you're really struggling, make sure you seek expert advice.

CARE FOR
YOUR PSYCHE...
KNOW THYSELF,
FOR ONCE
WE KNOW
OURSELVES,
WE MAY LEARN
HOW TO CARE
FOR OURSELVES.

SOCRATES

# Sleep Self-Care

Most of us have little time or energy to prepare our mind and body for a restorative night of sleep. Often we are so rushed that we delay sleeping to cram in all our daily commitments before we flop on to the sofa, exhausted. But it doesn't have to be this way – with a few small steps, you can help your mind and body prepare for better sleep. This will allow you to recover and let you wake up feeling refreshed to take on the day. Here is where the power of sleep self-care comes in. Read on to see how...

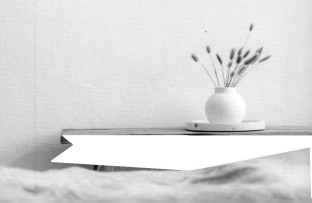

# SET A REGULAR BEDTIME

The sleep–wake cycle is part of your body clock over a 24-hour period. By following a regular bedtime and waking up at the same time every day, you are helping to keep this very important function in sync and reducing the risk of disruptive sleep.

Set a time you want to fall asleep and wake up. Use an old-fashioned alarm clock so you can keep phones and electronic devices in another room to prevent any scrolling urges.

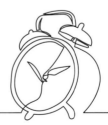

LIFE'S LITTLE
RITUALS CAN
TURN AN
ORDINARY
DAY INTO AN
EXTRAORDINARY
DAY –
**A RIGHT DAY.**

*Anonymous*

# ROUTINES AND RITUALS

We are creatures of comfort and our brains love predictability. This is why keeping weekly or daily routines and rituals is a perfect way to promote good quality-sleep for the restless mind and body.

The act of slowing down, taking time out from your busy schedule to read, meditate, bathe or do something restful helps you to unwind and recharge. Find what works for you, whether that's walking daily (page 42), setting a regular bedtime (page 107), having a mealtime ritual (page 67) or a weekend morning retreat (page 46) – it's entirely your choice. What small rituals can you bring into your schedule?

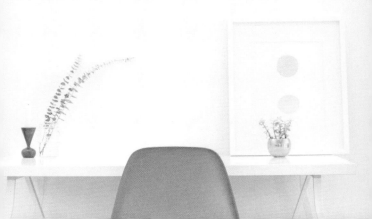

# FLOATING RITUAL

Rituals don't need to be elaborate, simply having a bath itself can be a ritual if you use the opportunity to truly relax and retreat. Research shows a hot bath an hour or two before bedtime decreases your body temperature by 1°C (1.8°F), which is the ideal temperature to fall asleep.

Studies confirm floating in water encourages restoration in the mind and body by simply disconnecting us from sensory stimulation.

Here's how to have a rest-inducing bath:

- Fill your bath with warm water. Light tea lights or candles around it and turn off any bright lights. Add a few drops of your favourite essential oils (page 113) or dissolve some Epsom salts to soothe aches and pains. Play some calming tunes to help you unwind. Undress mindfully – really slowing your movements down. Sprinkle a little sea salt on a damp facecloth and softly scrub your body, releasing the day's stresses. Float in the bath for 20 minutes and visualize bliss (page 57).

- Climb out of the bath slowly and dry yourself in towels or a fluffy bathrobe. Drink a replenishing herbal tea, such as peppermint, to replace fluid loss. Then, follow your bedtime routine, allowing yourself to truly let go of the day.

# SLEEPY SUPERFOODS

Many proteins, nutrients and hormones work together to promote good sleep and regulate your sleep cycle. Try eating foods which include sleep-friendly amino acids and minerals, such as potassium, tryptophan and magnesium, in the run-up to bedtime to help settle your mind and body. Almonds, walnuts, kiwis, oily fish, lettuce, cherries, blueberries and kale are just some of the foods that enhance sleep quality.

Research shows carotenoids, such as lutein, found in egg yolks, can improve your sleep too.

# ESSENTIAL OILS

Essential oils are marvellous for their powerful calming effect on our mood – and they're simple to use for sleep-promoting rituals. Of course, there are many essential oils, all with their own fragrances, so find ones that you're drawn to.

Try any of these super-effective oils: anxiety-relieving ylang-ylang, mood-lifting bergamot, mind-relaxing lavender, insomnia-soothing vetiver, stress-calming sweet orange, tension-releasing cedarwood, emotion-balancing geranium and tranquillizing chamomile.

Add a few drops to your bath, use diffuser sticks, sprinkle some droplets on your pillow or make a sleep-boosting pillow mist (page 134).

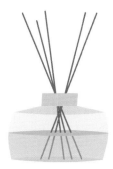

# Write a list

It's normal for pesky thoughts to run wild when you're trying to fall asleep. It happens to most of us from time to time because our minds are still active from a busy day.

One good way to quieten thoughts about all the things you need to do in the upcoming days is to get them out of your head and on to paper. This might seem a little strange right before bedtime, but by writing it down, you're offloading from your brain. Simply jot down your thoughts and put your list away. You will be able to tackle the list when you are refreshed and recharged.

Do not
anticipate trouble or
worry about what may
never happen. Keep in
the sunlight.

**BENJAMIN
FRANKLIN**

# LOCK AWAY WORRIES

If you're struggling to get that much-needed sleep because niggling worries are stirring up waves of emotion, fear not. It's quite normal for anxiety to peak at bedtime. A proven technique for negative thoughts is to imagine locking them away in a worry box and visualize putting the box under the bed.

Alongside this, try an exercise such as the body scan (page 60), muscle relaxation (page 74), breathing (pages 34 and 76), affirmations (page 125) or visualization (page 53) to help you drift off into a peaceful sleep.

# SIMPLE STRETCHES

Before you sleep, try these simple stretches to help you unwind and release tension:

- Gently stretch your arms up in the air, lower them slowly, massage your neck and shoulders, roll your head from side to side.

- Stretch your eyes by keeping them open, roll them slowly in a circular motion a few times in each direction. Close your eyes and repeat the eye-rolling.

- Finish by taking four deep breaths. Give yourself a bear hug by inhaling, opening your arms out wide and then crossing them over to give yourself a hug as you exhale.

# Restorative yoga

Restorative yoga is a remarkable practice that helps to soothe your mind and body. What makes it utterly wonderful is its power to calm the nervous system and encourage deep sleep. Studies show it can also relieve insomnia symptoms by activating your parasympathetic nervous system to settle your stress response. Try these yoga poses:

### Legs up the Wall

Lie on the floor and rest your legs against a wall at a 90-degree angle, using a cushion to support your back if needed. Twenty minutes of this pose can have the same restful benefits as a nap.

**Happy Baby**

Lying flat on the floor or on your bed, bend your knees toward your chest at a 90-degree angle and hold the inside of your feet, spreading your knees apart. Rock gently from side to side, mimicking a happy baby.

**Savasana**

Lying on your back in bed with your hands by your sides, allow your body to rest. Use pillows under your knees for support if required. Gently close your eyes, relax your shoulders, fill your belly with deep breaths, exhaling any tension and repeat until you float off to sleep.

Try combining these poses with the other exercises here or on page 66, or create your own yoga flow.

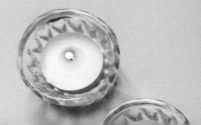

# HUG IN A MUG

There's a lot to be said about a comforting, warm drink to lull you into a state of zen before bedtime. Mothers knew what they were doing when they sent us to bed with a mug of warm milk, as some evidence suggests that upon drinking, tryptophan (an amino acid found in milk) is converted to melatonin, the hormone that regulates our natural sleep state.

Give yourself a comforting hug in a mug with these remedies:

- To drift off into a restful sleep, drink a mug of warm milk or almond milk. For added healing benefits try golden milk, which is brimming with nutrients that calm your breathing and relieve joint pain, fatigue and digestive issues.

- To make golden milk, combine 1 cup of milk, 1 tsp turmeric, 1 small piece of ginger (grated) and 1 tsp honey. Bring it to the boil, reduce the heat and simmer for 3 minutes. Strain if desired.

- Experiment with herbal teas such as decaffeinated green tea (proven to reduce stress) or mint. Super-calming chamomile tea is particularly helpful for people who suffer from insomnia.

# BE SCREEN-FREE

Many of us reach for our phones or tablets at bedtime, but unfortunately screens emit blue light which interferes with our production of melatonin, leading to disturbed sleep cycles.

Instead of stimulating your body and mind, reduce your exposure to blue light and help your body naturally prepare for sleep. By cutting out screens an hour before bedtime, you'll doze off more quickly, which will encourage deep restorative sleep throughout the night. To avoid screen temptations, leave your device in another room, read a book or listen to music instead.

This is a
wonderful day.
I have never seen
this one before.

MAYA ANGELOU

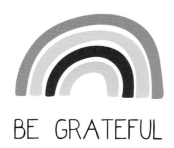

# BE GRATEFUL

Some research shows that gratitude promotes restorative sleep by improving mood, which leads to better and longer rest. Research also shows people who keep a gratitude journal may sleep 30 minutes more per night, wake up feeling more refreshed and experience more alertness during the day than those who don't.

Why not try jotting down three things you're grateful for before bedtime to help you get that good-quality shut-eye? Take a moment to reflect on all the good in your day. Add a gratitude ritual to your bedtime routine.

# AFFIRMATION RITUAL

Research tells us expecting to get a poor night's sleep can make falling asleep more difficult. Using positive sleep affirmations puts you in a more helpful mindset to welcome sound sleep.

Make positive affirmations a bedtime ritual. Try the ones here or write your own – go with whatever feels right. Read them aloud or repeat them in your head like a mantra as you lie in bed.

- I am relaxed and prepared for restorative sleep.

- I will sleep soundly.

- My bedroom is a sleep sanctuary.

- I deserve to sleep so I am recharged for tomorrow.

- I will wake feeling refreshed and alert.

# Soothing sounds

Soothing sounds are superb for relaxing your mind and body, especially if you are surrounded by noise throughout the day. In fact, studies show sound may play an essential role in your ability to doze off and stay asleep. Try these:

- Pink noise includes soothing nature sounds such as a trickling river, ocean waves or rainfall – these sounds promote deep sleep and enhance memory. Soundtracks are available on YouTube and elsewhere online.

- If your neighbours are loud or you live in a bustling city, play white noise to mute background sounds that might be preventing you from drifting off to sleep. White noise is available on sleep apps.

- Adding binaural beats to your playlist could give you auditory bliss. By offering specific tones and frequency in each ear, research shows that these beats can lessen anxious feelings and lull you to sleep. Numerous tracks are available online.

- Music can also encourage floating off into a deep sleep. Choose tracks that have 60 beats per minute or less because these are linked to elevating levels of deep restorative sleep.

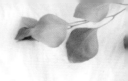

# TOASTY TOES

Research shows warming your feet for 20 minutes before bedtime can reduce symptoms of insomnia and fatigue. Wearing socks to bed can aid falling asleep faster and staying asleep longer. It also helps to lessen hot flushes and prevent cracked feet, especially when a healing skin lotion is applied to feet before covering with socks.

So if you're struggling to nod off, slip on a pair of cosy bed socks or slippers, try a nourishing foot massage, soak your feet in warm water or add a fluffy blanket to the end of your bed so you're pleasantly heated and comfy, ready for slumber.

# USE YOUR IMAGINATION

The way you think and what you think is proven to be a powerful tool in helping you drift off into the land of sweet dreams faster.

Visualize yourself doing an activity that you're good at. Perhaps imagine you're playing a musical instrument or cooking your favourite dish; let it be anything that makes you happy.

Make up a story – imagine something amazing is happening for you, such as landing your dream job or going on holiday in calming nature.

It also helps to imagine something wildly boring like counting every single grain of sand on a beach or peeling hundreds of carrots!

# IMAGINATION IS EVERYTHING.
IT IS THE PREVIEW OF LIFE'S COMING ATTRACTIONS.

ALBERT EINSTEIN

# Good Nights

We now have more distractions in the night than ever that upset our sleep—wake cycle, from the light from street lamps to cars driving past and phone screens. Although we might be achieving more, we're also sleeping less, with 62 per cent of adults globally saying they're not sleeping well. But by taking proactive steps, it is entirely possible to get the deep restorative sleep you need to feel refreshed and function healthily in all areas of your life – and it's surprisingly easy to do. Read on to tune in to the power of a good night's sleep.

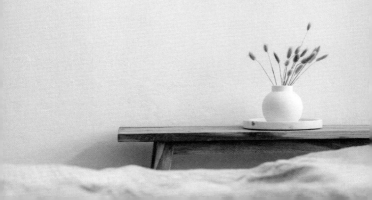

# CREATE A SLEEPING HAVEN

Does your bedroom make you feel calm or stressed? Your bedroom is your sleep haven and should bring you a sense of tranquillity. Here's how to boost your bedroom's zen ambience:

- Declutter messy shelves or drawers.

- Add flowers such as roses or lavender and sleep-friendly essential oils to encourage sweet dreams.

- Choose calming tones like blues or greens which relax your brain and soothe your nervous system.

- Use soft, gentle lighting – candles work beautifully (although always make sure these are extinguished before falling asleep). Pick ones made with essential oils and try blackout curtains or a sleep mask to avoid light disruption.

- Cultivate quiet (using earplugs or white noise).

- Keep your room at a comfortable temperature – ideally 18.3°C (65°F).

We shall
find renewal
in rest.

LAILAH GIFTY AKITA

# PILLOW TALK

Pillows aren't just for fluffing up and looking pretty, they need to be comfortable too. A poor pillow can undo all the rituals and preparation for sleep, and lead to aches and pains due to your spine not getting the proper support it needs.

Of course, pillows are a personal choice – your sleeping position, weight and anatomy can all affect how your pillow feels so it's worth finding one that meets your needs. For example, a snorer might need a higher pillow to keep their head elevated, while side sleepers might need a firm pillow for extra support.

Whichever pillow you go for, spray it with this easy-to-make dreamy pillow mist which will do wonders to entice you to sleep.

You will need:

- 1 measuring jug
- 1 small glass spray bottle
- 15 g (½ oz) witch hazel
- 60 ml (2 fl. oz) water
- 15 drops of lavender oil

**Method**

In the jug, mix the witch hazel and essential oils together, then add water. Now, pour the liquid mixture into the spray bottle. Shake and spritz over your pillow.

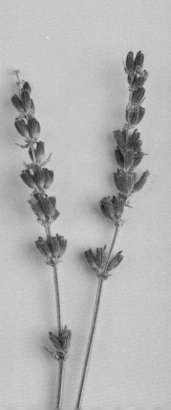

# GET COMFORTABLE BEDDING

Believe it or not, some research shows that your choice of bedding can affect your sleep. Freshly washed sheets create a sense of comfort which encourages rest. They also reduce dust mites. It's important to change your bedding to reflect seasonal temperatures, as being too hot or cold can disturb your sleep.

Don't forget about your mattress. If you're waking up with aches and pains or there are permanent dents in your mattress, it might be time to change it. It's recommended that bedding is replaced at least every five to eight years.

# COMFY
# NIGHTWEAR

Getting into loose, comfortable sleepwear can help you feel ready to switch off and relax. Make it your bedtime routine that once you're in comfy nightwear, it's time to wind down. Try not to look at any work emails or do anything stressful. Instead, start your bedtime rituals.

Try to avoid tight or itchy fabrics – choose loose, lightweight cotton pyjamas for warmer temperatures and cosy flannel ones during winter.

# KNOW YOUR SLUMBER POSE

Most of us have a favourite sleeping position, whether that's lying on our front, side or back. As soon as you get under the sheets, it's helpful to strike your best sleep pose immediately as this lessens the chance of restlessness when you're drifting off into the early stages of sleep.

Ideally, your sleep position should promote healthy spinal alignment from your hips to your head. Sleeping on your side or back is considered beneficial; however, if sleeping on your front feels great, don't feel pressured to change it – you can enhance spinal alignment with the right pillow and mattress.

# SOOTHE INSOMNIA

Some studies show acupressure can help to relieve insomnia. In fact, simply using the pressure of your fingers and thumbs to stimulate acupressure points can be a remarkable way to soothe your emotions. Try this:

- Place a finger behind each earlobe, tilt your head back and you should find a small hollow behind the bony ridge. Apply pressure for 30 seconds to clear your head.

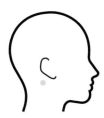

- Bend your hand forward to find the crease on your inner wrist. Apply pressure to the outermost point of this crease, on the side closest to your little finger for a minute to feel calmer.

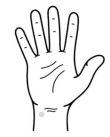

SHOOT FOR
THE MOON.
EVEN IF YOU
MISS, YOU'LL
LAND AMONG
THE STARS.

*Norman Vincent Peale*

# REFRAME NEGATIVE THOUGHTS

Sometimes we lie awake tossing and turning, telling ourselves, "I must get eight hours of sleep, I won't be able to function tomorrow," or "Insomnia is going to make me ill." These thoughts are not facts and make it so much harder to fall asleep. Thankfully, reframing them can help you drift off and deal with insomnia. Every time a negative thought pops up, replace it with a positive sleep thought such as, "I can relax and sleep, falling asleep is easy and natural for me." Do this any time you notice negative sleep thoughts.

# Insomnia-busting remedies

Natural remedies can be game-changing. Try valerian, an anxiety-reducing and sleep-improving herbal remedy which you can brew as tea or take as a supplement. For added healing benefits, combine valerian with lemon balm to help induce sleepiness and slow your breathing. Drink a cup of valerian and lemon balm tea an hour before bed. Teabags are available online and in grocery stores.

Studies show using eye masks or earplugs may help you to fall asleep quicker and get quality shut-eye, as well

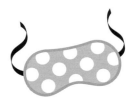

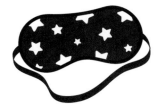

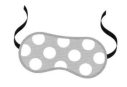

as improve your ability to sleep in noisier surroundings. Choose an eye mask made with breathable material and adjustable straps, ensuring it feels gentle on your skin and completely blocks out all light. The most practical choices might not win any style points, but that's okay!

Why not use a thin muslin cloth or cotton fabric to make pillow sachets full of dried lavender? Place these fragrant sachets inside your pillowcase, under your pillow or in your linen cupboard for freshly scented sheets to help you doze off.

Tart cherry juice increases your body's production of melatonin and has been shown to ease insomnia when drunk daily for two weeks. Try this nutrient-rich juice to help you drift off to a restful sleep.

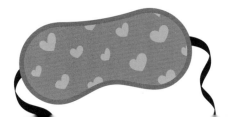

# BREATHE AWAY SLEEPLESSNESS

We all experience insomnia at some point, but you don't have to put up with endless sleepless nights. When you find yourself wide awake and restless with despair in the early hours, let breathing and relaxation techniques be your go-to answer. Breathe in through your nose for four counts, hold your breath for seven counts, then exhale through your mouth for eight counts. This triggers the parasympathetic nervous system and slows your heart rate to help you float off into a lovely deep sleep.

You could also try autogenic training, a relaxation technique which stops anxiety in its tracks. It's similar to scanning your body but adds statements about the warmth and heaviness as you focus on each part of your body, to help calm you. Start by noticing your breathing for a minute. Then bring your awareness to your feet and say, "My feet are warm, I am calm." Repeat five times. Next say, "My feet are heavy, I am calm." Repeat five times. Do this for your hands, shoulders, back and head to doze off. For further instructions, download autogenic training audios or try any of the breathing exercises in this book.

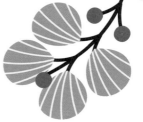

# GET YOUR ROUTINE RIGHT

Getting good-quality sleep is an all-day event. Try getting up when the alarm buzzes instead of snoozing, then eat a healthy breakfast and get outdoors for daylight exposure. This will set your body and mind up for a good day, which will have a positive impact on the quality of your sleep.

Stick to regular mealtimes and try to avoid poor food choices that are high in sugar or heavily processed as these will cause energy slumps. Opt for sleep-promoting foods (page 112) instead. Avoid large heavy meals before bedtime as it's harder to fall asleep when your body is still digesting food. Why not introduce an evening mealtime ritual (page 67) containing light and healthy meals?

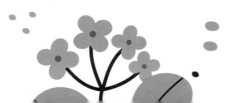

# BE MINDFUL OF YOUR WORKOUT

Daily exercise is beneficial for your health, but when it comes to sleep, it's important to time it right. Sleep experts recommend avoiding intense workouts close to bedtime because they can spoil your body's capacity to settle down before sleep. So if you are going to exercise, allow your body enough time to return to its natural resting state before heading to bed.

Research suggests moderate-intensity exercises, such as yoga, stretching, walking or swimming, within 60 to 90 minutes of bedtime do not affect sleep negatively. Be mindful of your workout so you can pick times and exercises that won't disrupt your sleep.

# SET SLEEP BOUNDARIES

Sleep is vital for your mental and physical well-being, so that you can function better in all areas of your life. Maintaining good sleep is hugely important, but with so many demands and distractions coming from family, work and life, it's not always easy to do. This is where setting sleep boundaries comes in.

First and foremost, reserve your bed for sleep and sex only. You might be tempted to work on your bed with your laptop, but this doesn't help your brain associate your bed with sleep and may keep you awake

If you share a household with your family or partner, it's essential that everyone is aware that sleep is a priority. Set consistent sleep–wake times for everyone.

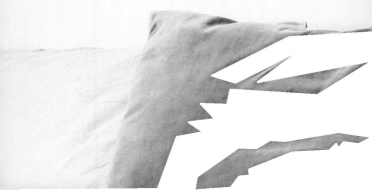

Be mindful of pets as, while they can be calming and great companions, if you're a light sleeper or are having sleep troubles because of your mental health, you might want to keep your furry friends off your bed or out of your bedroom altogether.

If you have a restless partner who scrolls on their phone or snacks in bed, tell them about the importance of good sleep self-care and see if they'll change some of their bad habits – you'll both sleep better!

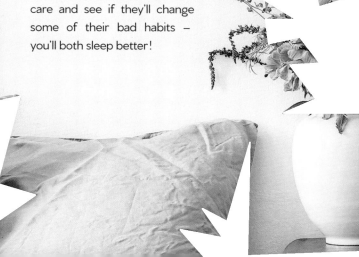

# BE NAP-WISE

A daytime nap can offer a much-needed energy boost to tackle the day, especially if you're sleep-deprived. But it's essential to get the timing and length of naps right to avoid disrupting your sleep. Ideally, a nap lasting between 10 and 20 minutes prevents you from falling into deeper sleep phases and waking up groggy.

Studies show the best time to nap is early to mid-afternoon – around 2 p.m. So go ahead, take that restorative nap wisely and should you feel befuddled upon waking, splash cold water on your face and sip a body-boosting juice, leaving you ready to take on the rest of the day.

# Break the cycle

When you find yourself lying awake after trying for a long time to fall asleep, it's helpful to actually get up. By staying in bed, your mind associates your bed with sleeplessness and frustration.

To avoid this unhealthy cycle, after 20 minutes of lying awake, get out of bed to do something in dim light that will help you chill. Try to take your mind off sleep — perhaps try a breathing exercise, visualization or sleep affirmations to help you reset. Once you're ready, try going to sleep again.

# BE MINDFUL OF SLEEPING PILLS

Many people use sleeping pills for quick relief to ease short-term stress such as that from a traumatic situation, jet lag or a temporary issue that's disturbing their sleep. While some sleeping pills help you fall asleep, others aid staying asleep and some do both.

Be aware that regular use of sleeping medication can create dependency and many of the side effects are unpleasant. This is why it's essential to be mindful before taking sleeping pills and to discuss the risks and benefits with your doctor.

# AND SUDDENLY YOU JUST KNOW IT'S TIME
## TO START SOMETHING NEW AND TRUST THE MAGIC OF BEGINNINGS.

MEISTER ECKHART

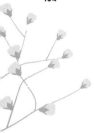

# CONCLUSION

The power of rest is so important to each one of us. Hopefully, this book has helped you to create more respite in your daily life so you feel refreshed and recharged, ready to tackle each day at your best. Building healthy habits can take a little time – whether it's setting a bedtime routine, getting outdoors for a daily walk or carving out space in your schedule to take care of your rest needs. Remember – by taking those first small proactive steps, you'll be restoring your mind and body and setting yourself up for brighter days.

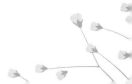

Now all you need to do is stay focused on your rest
needs and maintain your boundaries. Don't feel guilty
for taking time to recharge and try not to fill your rest
time with more work or scrolling online. Give yourself
permission to recharge your batteries. Allow yourself to
savour those moments of downtime as they will leave
you feeling energized, happier and more relaxed across
all areas of your life. Rest matters, you matter and those
around you deserve you at your best. So, slow down
and enjoy the power of rest. You totally deserve it.

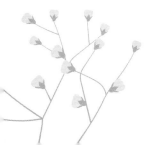

# Image credits

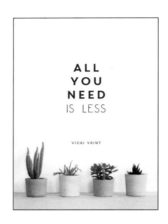

### *All You Need Is Less*
### Vicki Vrint
### Hardback
### 978-1-78685-766-8

This little book, filled with practical tips and ideas, covers a range of topics, including how to stress less, reduce screen time, minimize clutter, shop sustainably and make the most of your "me" time. By choosing a lifestyle that is less busy, less cluttered and less stressful, you will instantly feel healthier and happier.

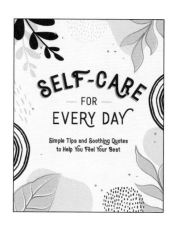

*Self-Care for Every Day*
**Hardback**
**978-1-80007-674-7**

Discover the joy of self-care with the help of this beautiful little book. Including self-care inspiration to nourish your mind, body and soul, advice on fitting self-care into a busy schedule, and a raft of soothing quotes, it will help you to nurture your well-being every day.

Have you enjoyed this book?
If so, find us on Facebook at **Summersdale
Publishers**, on Twitter at **@Summersdale**
and on Instagram at **@summersdalebooks** and
get in touch. We'd love to hear from you!

## www.summersdale.com